NUTRITION FOR LONGEVITY:

Burn Fat, Restore Metabolism, And Thrive.

Victor T. Rice

INTRODUCTION 5

CHAPTER 1 10

UNDERSTANDING LONGEVITY NUTRITION 10

What is Longevity Nutrition? 10

The Impact of Diet on Longevity 11

Key Components of Longevity Nutrition....................11

The Basics of Metabolic Processes 15

Factors Influencing Metabolism................................15

Metabolism and Aging 16

CHAPTER 3 18

THE SCIENCE OF FAT BURNING............................18

Understanding the Dynamics of Fat Metabolism 18

Types of Fat and Their Roles....................................18

Strategies to Optimize Fat Burning 20

CHAPTER 4 22

EXERCISE AND METABOLISM 22

Exercise as a Catalyst for Metabolic Health 22

Best Exercise Practices for Fat Burning....................23

Combining Nutrition and Exercise for Maximum Results ..24

CHAPTER 5 26

MACRONUTRIENTS AND LONGEVITY 26

Understanding Carbohydrates, Proteins, and Fats 26

Balancing Macronutrients for Longevity 27

Impact of Macronutrient Ratios on Health span 28

CHAPTER 6 30

MICRONUTRIENTS AND LONGEVITY 30

Essential Micronutrients for Longevity 30

The Role of Micronutrients in Health and Longevity 31

Sources and Optimal Intake of Micronutrients 32

CHAPTER 7 34

SUPERFOODS AND LONGEVITY 34

Exploring Nature's Powerhouses 34

Incorporating Superfoods into Your Diet 35

Unveiling the Health Benefits 36

CHAPTER 8 38

INTERMITTENT FASTING AND LONGEVITY 38

Understanding Intermittent Fasting 38

Benefits and Potential Impact on Health span 39

Implementing Intermittent Fasting Safely 40

CHAPTER 9 42

STRESS MANAGEMENT AND LONGEVITY 42

Understanding the Impact of Stress on Health 42

Stress Reduction Techniques and Practices 43

Creating a Stress-Resilient Lifestyle 43

CHAPTER 10 45

SLEEP AND LONGEVITY 45

Importance of Quality Sleep 45

Factors Influencing Sleep Quality 46

Tips for Improving Sleep Quality and Duration 46

CHAPTER 11 48

PERSONALIZED NUTRITION FOR LONGEVITY 48

Understanding Personalized Nutrition 48

Approaches to Personalization 49

Implementing Personalized Nutrition Strategies.................49

CHAPTER 12 51

LONGEVITY MINDSET AND LIFESTYLE
INTEGRATION 51

The Power of Mindset in Longevity 51

Holistic Lifestyle Integration 52

Implementing Lifestyle Habits for Longevity 53

CHAPTER 13: 55

SUSTAINABLE PRACTICES FOR LONG-TERM 55

HEALTH 55

Consistency in Healthy Habits....................................55

Overcoming Roadblocks to Sustainability 56

Longevity in Lifestyle Integration 57

CONCLUSION 59

INTRODUCTION

Welcome to "Nutrition for Longevity: Burn Fat, Restore Metabolism, and Thrive." In an era where the pursuit of longevity and vibrant health takes center stage, understanding the pivotal role of nutrition in achieving these goals becomes paramount. This book is your comprehensive guide, designed to unravel the intricate relationship between what you eat, how your body functions, and its profound impact on your lifespan and well-being.

The quest for optimal health span often feels like navigating a maze in the bustling landscape of fad diets, quick fixes, and ever-evolving health trends. Amidst this confusion, this book serves as a beacon of clarity, offering evidence-based insights, practical strategies, and a holistic approach to nutrition tailored explicitly for longevity.

Unveiling the Core Principles

Within these pages, we delve deep into the core principles of longevity nutrition, meticulously exploring the intricate workings of your metabolism, the science of fat burning, and the profound influence of macronutrients and micronutrients on your body's longevity potential. But this isn't merely a theoretical exploration; it's a roadmap—a journey through the intricate pathways of your body's systems, unveiling how your food choices impact your metabolism, cellular health, and overall vitality.

Beyond Diet: Lifestyle Factors for Longevity

Nutrition, however, is just one piece of the puzzle. Recognizing the significance of lifestyle factors, we'll also venture into intermittent fasting, stress management techniques, the crucial role of quality sleep, and the harmonious integration of exercise into your life—each playing a pivotal role in the grand symphony of longevity.

Personalized Approach to Longevity

Understanding that each individual is unique, we'll guide you in tailoring a personalized longevity diet plan, emphasizing sustainability and adaptability. With practical tips, meal plans, and recipes, this book aims to educate and empower you to make informed choices and transform your relationship with food and lifestyle.

Embracing a Longevity Mindset

Lastly, this book advocates for more than just dietary changes; it champions a mindset shift—a commitment to your long-term health and well-being. Through actionable steps, case studies, and guidance, we aim to inspire a mindset that transcends short-term fixes, fostering a lifestyle deeply rooted in the pursuit of vitality and longevity.

Let's Begin the Journey

Join us as we embark on this enlightening voyage through the realms of nutrition, metabolism, and lifestyle, aimed not just at adding years to your life but adding life to your years. Together, let's unlock the secrets of longevity and nutrition, fuel our bodies optimally, and thrive in the pursuit of a healthier, happier, and more vibrant life.

CHAPTER 1

UNDERSTANDING LONGEVITY NUTRITION

The Pursuit of Longevity

In a world where the quest for longevity and vibrant health occupies the collective consciousness, the significance of nutrition stands as a cornerstone. Longevity nutrition isn't merely about extending the years you spend on this planet; it's about enhancing the quality of those years, ensuring vitality, resilience, and well-being throughout your life's journey.

What is Longevity Nutrition?

Longevity nutrition encompasses a deliberate, strategic approach to food choices and dietary habits that extend beyond basic sustenance. It revolves around selecting and consuming foods that optimize your body's functions, preserve cellular health, and promote vitality, thereby enhancing your potential for a longer, healthier life.

The Impact of Diet on Longevity

Scientific research continues to reaffirm the powerful influence of diet on the aging process and overall health span. Certain dietary patterns rich in whole foods, antioxidants, and essential nutrients can mitigate the risk of chronic diseases, improve metabolic health, and potentially slow down the aging process at a cellular level.

Key Components of Longevity Nutrition

Longevity nutrition isn't a one-size-fits-all paradigm; rather, it's a multifaceted approach that encompasses various key components:

- Nutrient Density:

Emphasizing foods rich in essential vitamins, minerals, antioxidants, and phytonutrients that nourish the body at a cellular level and support optimal function.

- Balanced Macronutrients:

Understanding the role of carbohydrates, proteins, and fats in the body and achieving a balanced intake to support metabolic health and energy production.

- Mindful Eating:

Cultivating awareness and conscious eating practices, such as mindful eating, which involves paying attention to hunger cues, savoring flavors, and being present during meals.

- Quality and Sources of Food:

Prioritize whole, unprocessed foods over highly refined or ultra-processed options, and consider factors such as food sourcing, organic choices, and sustainable practices.

- Individualization:

Acknowledging that individual needs, preferences, and genetic factors play a crucial role in determining the most suitable approach to nutrition for each person's longevity journey.

Navigating the Path Forward

In this chapter, we've scratched the surface of the expansive realm of longevity nutrition, outlining its fundamental principles and highlighting its profound impact on health and longevity. As we progress through this book, we'll delve deeper into specific aspects of nutrition, metabolism, and lifestyle practices, equipping you with the knowledge and tools necessary to optimize your dietary choices and foster a healthier, more vibrant life.

Join us on this enlightening journey as we unravel the mysteries of longevity nutrition and discover the transformative power of food and lifestyle choices in the pursuit of a longer, healthier life.

CHAPTER 2
METABOLISM DEMYSTIFIED

Exploring the Body's Energy Machinery

Metabolism, the sum of biochemical processes within the body, intricately governs how energy is produced and utilized. Understanding its mechanisms is pivotal in optimizing health and longevity. In this chapter, we delve deep into the fundamental aspects of metabolism, unraveling its complexities and shedding light on its significance in the pursuit of a healthier life.

The Basics of Metabolic Processes

Metabolism involves an array of processes that convert food into energy, supporting bodily functions such as cell repair, growth, and movement. At its core, metabolism encompasses two primary processes:

- Catabolism:

The breakdown of larger molecules into smaller units releases energy that the body can use.

- Anabolism:

The synthesis of complex molecules from simpler ones requires energy for cellular growth and repair.

Factors Influencing Metabolism

Various factors influence an individual's metabolic rate, impacting how efficiently the body utilizes energy:

- Basal Metabolic Rate (BMR):

The energy expended while at rest to maintain basic physiological functions like breathing and circulation. Factors such as age, gender, body composition, and genetics influence BMR.

- Hormonal Regulation:

Hormones like insulin, thyroid hormones, and cortisol play critical roles in regulating metabolic processes and influencing energy expenditure and storage.

- Physical Activity and Exercise:

The level and type of physical activity significantly impact metabolism, affecting calorie expenditure and fat utilization.

Metabolism and Aging

As individuals age, metabolic processes undergo changes. BMR tends to decrease, and hormonal fluctuations may occur, affecting metabolic efficiency. Understanding these age-related shifts in metabolism becomes imperative in adopting strategies to maintain metabolic health and vitality as one grows older.

Navigating Metabolic Health

This chapter offers a foundational understanding of metabolism—its core processes and the multitude of factors that shape its functionality. By comprehending how the body's energy machinery operates, you gain valuable insights into how dietary and lifestyle choices can influence metabolic health. Armed with this knowledge, you'll be better equipped to optimize your metabolism, paving the way for enhanced energy levels, improved health, and potentially extending your health span.

In the subsequent chapters, we'll further explore how the science of metabolism intertwines with nutrition, exercise, and lifestyle, providing you with actionable strategies to harness the power of metabolic health in your pursuit of longevity.

CHAPTER 3
THE SCIENCE OF FAT BURNING

Understanding the Dynamics of Fat Metabolism

Fat, an essential component of the human body, serves as an energy store and plays a crucial role in various physiological functions. In this chapter, we'll unravel the intricate science behind fat metabolism, explore how the body processes and utilizes fats, and unveil strategies to optimize fat burning for improved health and longevity.

Types of Fat and Their Roles

- Saturated, Unsaturated, and Trans Fats:
Different types of fats have varying effects on health. Understanding the distinctions between these fats is vital for making informed dietary choices.

- **Brown Fat vs. White Fat:**

Delving into the distinction between brown and white fat, elucidating their roles in metabolism, energy expenditure, and potential implications for weight management.

Mechanisms of Fat Metabolism

- **Lipolysis:**

The breakdown of stored fat into fatty acids and glycerol, which are then utilized for energy production or stored for future use.

- **Ketosis:**

Exploring the metabolic state of ketosis, where the body predominantly uses fat for fuel instead of carbohydrates, and its relevance in fat burning and weight management.

Strategies to Optimize Fat Burning

- Balanced Nutrition:

Adopting a balanced diet that supports fat metabolism by including healthy fats, lean proteins, and complex carbohydrates in appropriate proportions.

- Physical Activity and Exercise:

Engaging in regular physical activity and exercise routines that promote fat burning and contribute to overall metabolic health.

- Intermittent Fasting:

Exploring intermittent fasting as a strategy to enhance fat metabolism and improve metabolic flexibility.

Harnessing the Power of Fat Metabolism

Understanding the science behind fat metabolism provides valuable insights into how dietary and lifestyle choices impact the body's ability to burn fat for energy.

By adopting evidence-based strategies outlined in this chapter, you'll be empowered to optimize fat metabolism, support weight management, enhance energy levels, and potentially contribute to overall health and longevity.
In the subsequent chapters, we'll further explore the synergistic relationship between fat metabolism, nutrition, and lifestyle factors, providing actionable insights to help you harness the power of fat metabolism for a healthier, more vibrant life.

CHAPTER 4
EXERCISE AND METABOLISM

Exploring the Symbiotic Relationship

Exercise stands as a cornerstone in the pursuit of optimal metabolic health and fat burning. In this chapter, we'll delve into the intricate relationship between exercise and metabolism, elucidating how physical activity influences metabolic processes, supports fat-burning, and contributes to overall health and longevity.

Exercise as a Catalyst for Metabolic Health

- Impact on Metabolic Rate:

Understanding how different types of exercise influence the basal metabolic rate contributes to increased calorie expenditure and metabolic efficiency.

- Muscle Mass and Metabolism:

Exploring the connection between muscle mass, exercise, and metabolism, highlighting the role of muscle tissue in boosting metabolic rate and fat burning.

Best Exercise Practices for Fat Burning

- Aerobic Exercise vs. Strength Training: Comparing the effects of aerobic exercises (such as running or cycling) and strength training (weight lifting, resistance exercises) on fat metabolism and overall metabolic health.

- High-Intensity Interval Training (HIIT): Unveiling the potential benefits of HIIT, a form of exercise that alternates between intense bursts of activity and short rest periods, in enhancing fat burning and metabolic adaptation.

**Combining Nutrition and Exercise for Maximum
Results**
- Nutrient Timing:

Exploring how strategic nutrient timing, such as
consuming specific macronutrients before or after
exercise, can optimize fat metabolism and support
recovery.

- Synergistic Effects of Diet and Exercise:

Understanding how a balanced diet, when combined with
appropriate exercise routines, can synergistically enhance
metabolic health and fat burning.

Cultivating a Sustainable Exercise Routine

The chapter emphasizes the importance of finding an
exercise routine that aligns with individual preferences,
abilities, and lifestyle. By incorporating regular physical
activity into daily life and understanding its profound
effects on metabolism, you can harness the power of

exercise to support fat burning, improve metabolic health, and pave the way towards a longer, healthier life.

In the subsequent chapters, we'll continue to explore the interplay between nutrition, exercise, and metabolic health, providing actionable strategies to optimize these factors for enhanced vitality and longevity.

CHAPTER 5

MACRONUTRIENTS AND LONGEVITY

Balancing the Building Blocks of Nutrition

Macronutrients—carbohydrates, proteins, and fats—are the fundamental components of our diet, each playing a crucial role in supporting bodily functions and overall health. In this chapter, we'll explore the significance of macronutrients in longevity nutrition, understanding their roles, and achieving a balanced intake for optimal health span.

Understanding Carbohydrates, Proteins, and Fats

- Carbohydrates:

Exploring the various forms of carbohydrates, their impact on energy levels, and how they affect metabolism and blood sugar regulation.

- Proteins:

Unveiling the importance of proteins in supporting muscle health, cellular repair, and their role as building blocks for enzymes and hormones.

- **Fats:**
Examining the diverse types of dietary fats and understanding their roles in hormone production, cell membrane structure, and energy storage.

Balancing Macronutrients for Longevity

- **The Role of Balanced Nutrition:**
Emphasizing the significance of consuming a balanced ratio of macronutrients to support metabolic health, energy production, and overall well-being.

Impact of Macronutrient Ratios on Health span:

Investigating the effects of different macronutrient ratios on health, metabolism, and their potential implications for longevity.

Fine-Tuning Your Macronutrient Intake

- Personalized Approaches:

Acknowledging individual variations and the importance of tailoring macronutrient intake based on factors such as age, activity level, and metabolic needs.

- Strategies for Achieving Balance:

Providing practical tips and guidelines for achieving a well-rounded macronutrient intake through mindful food choices and portion control.

Integrating Longevity Nutrition Principles

Understanding the pivotal roles of carbohydrates, proteins, and fats in longevity nutrition enables you to make informed dietary choices that support optimal health and vitality. By balancing macronutrients and recognizing their impact on metabolic health, you lay the groundwork for a sustainable approach to nutrition that contributes to a longer, healthier life.

In the subsequent chapters, we'll continue to explore the multifaceted aspects of nutrition for longevity, delving deeper into micronutrients, superfoods, and personalized dietary approaches.

CHAPTER 6

MICRONUTRIENTS AND LONGEVITY

Exploring the Vital Components of Health and Longevity

Micronutrients, encompassing essential vitamins and minerals, are critical for maintaining overall health, supporting cellular function, and contributing to longevity. In this chapter, we'll delve into the significance of micronutrients in the pursuit of a balanced and sustainable diet for a longer, healthier life.

Essential Micronutrients for Longevity

- Vitamins:

Investigating the role of various vitamins, such as A, B, C, D, E, and K, in supporting immune function, tissue repair, and overall health.

- Minerals:

Understanding the importance of essential minerals like calcium, magnesium, iron, zinc, and others in maintaining bone health, energy production, and enzymatic functions.

The Role of Micronutrients in Health and Longevity

- Antioxidants and Aging:
Exploring the impact of antioxidants on neutralizing free radicals, oxidative stress, and their potential role in slowing down the aging process.

- Immune Function and Micronutrients:
Investigating how micronutrients play a crucial role in supporting immune system function, promoting resilience against infections, and aiding in recovery.

Sources and Optimal Intake of Micronutrients

- Dietary Sources:

Identifying natural food sources rich in vitamins and minerals and understanding the importance of diversity in the diet for micronutrient intake.

- Supplementation Considerations:

Discussing the role of supplements in filling potential nutrient gaps and considerations for their use in conjunction with a balanced diet.

Implementing Micronutrient-Rich Diets for Longevity

Understanding the significance of micronutrients empowers individuals to make informed dietary choices that prioritize the intake of vitamins and minerals essential for overall health and longevity. By embracing a diet rich in micronutrients, you lay the groundwork for enhanced cellular function, improved immune response, and potentially extended health span.

In the subsequent chapters, we'll continue to explore additional aspects of nutrition for longevity, including the incorporation of superfoods and practical strategies for implementing a personalized longevity-focused diet.

CHAPTER 7
SUPERFOODS AND LONGEVITY

Exploring Nature's Powerhouses

Superfoods, known for their exceptional nutritional density and health-promoting properties, have gained recognition for their potential contributions to longevity and overall well-being. In this chapter, we'll explore the world of superfoods, understand their benefits, incorporate them into diets, and maximize their potential for a healthier, longer life.

Understanding Superfoods

- Defining Superfoods:

Explore the concept of superfoods and identify key characteristics that categorize certain foods as superfoods due to their exceptional nutrient content.

- Diverse Range of Superfoods:

Highlighting various superfoods such as berries, leafy greens, nuts, seeds, oily fish, and others, and elucidating their specific nutritional profiles and health benefits.

Incorporating Superfoods into Your Diet

- Nutrient-Rich Additions:
Discussing ways to integrate superfoods into daily meals and snacks to enhance nutritional intake and promote overall health.

- Recipes and Ideas:
Providing practical recipes and creative ideas for incorporating superfoods into diverse and enjoyable dishes, encouraging variety and culinary exploration.

Unveiling the Health Benefits

- Antioxidant Properties:

Investigating how antioxidants present in many superfoods contribute to reducing oxidative stress, supporting cellular health, and potentially slowing down the aging process.

- Anti-Inflammatory Effects:

Exploring the potential of certain superfoods to possess anti-inflammatory properties, aiding in the prevention of chronic inflammation-related diseases.

Embracing Superfoods for Longevity

Understanding the potency of superfoods empowers individuals to optimize their nutritional intake, promoting overall health and potentially contributing to an extended health span. By incorporating a variety of nutrient-dense superfoods into a balanced diet, you pave the way for enhanced well-being and longevity.

In the subsequent chapters, we'll continue our exploration, discussing lifestyle strategies and practical implementations that complement the integration of superfoods into a comprehensive approach for longevity.

CHAPTER 8
INTERMITTENT FASTING AND LONGEVITY

Harnessing the Power of Fasting for Health span

Intermittent fasting, a dietary approach involving alternating cycles of eating and fasting, has garnered attention for its potential benefits on metabolic health, weight management, and potentially extending lifespan. In this chapter, we'll explore intermittent fasting as a strategy for longevity, examining its mechanisms, variations, and potential implications for health.

Understanding Intermittent Fasting

- **Fasting Patterns:**

Exploring different intermittent fasting protocols, such as the 16/8 method, alternate-day fasting, and time-restricted feeding, and understanding their structures and potential benefits.

- **Metabolic Effects:**

Investigating how intermittent fasting influences metabolic processes, such as insulin sensitivity, cellular repair mechanisms, and autophagy, potentially contributing to longevity.

Benefits and Potential Impact on Health span

- Weight Management:

Discussing the role of intermittent fasting in supporting weight loss, regulating appetite, and potentially improving body composition.

- Metabolic Health:

Examining the effects of intermittent fasting on metabolic markers, including blood sugar levels, cholesterol, and inflammation, and their implications for overall health.

Implementing Intermittent Fasting Safely

- **Tips for Success:**

Providing practical tips, strategies, and guidelines for implementing intermittent fasting safely and effectively, considering individual needs and potential challenges.

- **Potential Considerations:**

Discussing considerations for specific populations, such as pregnant individuals, individuals with certain medical conditions, and athletes, regarding the adoption of intermittent fasting.

Embracing Intermittent Fasting for Longevity

Understanding the potential benefits and considerations of intermittent fasting empowers individuals to explore this dietary approach as a tool for optimizing health and potentially extending their health span. By incorporating intermittent fasting in a safe and personalized manner, individuals can harness its potential benefits to support overall well-being.

In the subsequent chapters, we'll continue our exploration of lifestyle strategies and practical implementations that complement the pursuit of longevity through nutrition and wellness practices.

CHAPTER 9

STRESS MANAGEMENT AND LONGEVITY

Nurturing Resilience for a Longer, Healthier Life

Stress, a ubiquitous part of modern life, profoundly impacts health and well-being. In this chapter, we'll explore the intricate relationship between stress and longevity, examining the effects of stress on the body, strategies for managing stress, and fostering resilience for a healthier, more vibrant life.

Understanding the Impact of Stress on Health

- Physiological Response:

Exploring the body's stress response, including the role of cortisol and its impact on various bodily systems, such as the immune, cardiovascular, and digestive systems.

- Chronic Stress and Health Risks:

Investigating the potential implications of chronic stress on health, including increased susceptibility to diseases, inflammation, and accelerated aging processes.

Stress Reduction Techniques and Practices

- Mindfulness and Meditation:
Exploring mindfulness practices and meditation as tools to reduce stress, enhance emotional resilience, and promote overall well-being.

- Breathing Exercises and Relaxation Techniques:
Discussing the benefits of deep breathing exercises, progressive muscle relaxation, and other relaxation techniques in alleviating stress and tension.

Creating a Stress-Resilient Lifestyle

- Lifestyle Modifications:
Examining lifestyle factors that contribute to stress resilience, including adequate sleep, regular physical activity, and fostering social connections.

- **Coping Strategies:**

Providing practical coping strategies for managing stress, such as time management, setting boundaries, and prioritizing self-care practices.

Embracing Stress Management for Longevity

Understanding the impact of stress on health and adopting effective stress management techniques empowers individuals to proactively mitigate its detrimental effects. By incorporating stress-reducing practices into daily life, individuals can foster resilience, support overall health, and potentially enhance longevity.

In the subsequent chapters, we'll continue our exploration, discussing additional lifestyle strategies and practical implementations to promote a longer, healthier life through nutrition and wellness practices.

CHAPTER 10
SLEEP AND LONGEVITY

Embracing Quality Sleep for Health and Vitality

Sleep, an often overlooked yet essential aspect of health, plays a pivotal role in supporting overall well-being and longevity. In this chapter, we'll explore the significance of quality sleep, its impact on health, strategies for improving sleep quality, and its relationship to a longer, healthier life.

Importance of Quality Sleep

- Sleep Cycles and Stages:

Understanding the different stages of sleep, including REM (rapid eye movement) and non-REM sleep, and their contributions to restorative rest.

- Health Implications of Poor Sleep:

Investigating the potential health consequences of inadequate sleep, including impacts on cognitive function, immune health, and increased risk for chronic conditions.

Factors Influencing Sleep Quality
- Sleep Hygiene:

Discussing the importance of sleep hygiene practices, such as maintaining a consistent sleep schedule, creating a conducive sleep environment, and limiting exposure to electronic devices before bedtime.

- Stress and Sleep:

Exploring the relationship between stress, anxiety, and sleep quality, and strategies for managing stress to improve sleep.

Tips for Improving Sleep Quality and Duration

- Healthy Sleep Habits:

Providing practical tips for establishing healthy sleep habits, including relaxation techniques, bedtime rituals, and dietary considerations that support better sleep.

- **Addressing Sleep Disorders:**

Highlighting common sleep disorders such as insomnia and sleep apnea and offering guidance on seeking professional help for diagnosis and treatment.

Prioritizing Quality Sleep for Longevity

Recognizing the significance of quality sleep in supporting overall health and vitality empowers individuals to prioritize restorative rest as a pillar of longevity. By implementing healthy sleep practices and addressing factors that hinder sleep quality, individuals can promote better sleep, enhance well-being, and potentially extend their health span.

In the subsequent chapters, we'll continue our exploration, discussing additional lifestyle strategies and practical implementations for fostering a longer, healthier life through nutrition and wellness practices.

CHAPTER 11

PERSONALIZED NUTRITION FOR LONGEVITY

Tailoring Dietary Approaches to Individual Needs

Recognizing that each person is unique, with distinct nutritional requirements and preferences, personalized nutrition stands as a cornerstone for optimizing health span. In this chapter, we'll explore the principles and strategies behind personalized nutrition, considering individual needs, genetic variations, and lifestyle factors in crafting dietary approaches for longevity.

Understanding Personalized Nutrition

- Genetic Variability:

Exploring the impact of genetics on nutrient metabolism, preferences, and individual responses to dietary components.

- Metabolic Variations:

Investigating how factors like age, gender, activity level, and metabolic health influence individual nutritional needs.

Approaches to Personalization

- **Nutrigenomics and Nutrigenetics:**
Discussing the emerging fields of nutrigenomics and nutrigenetics, which study the interaction between genes, nutrition, and health outcomes.

- **Functional Testing:**
Exploring the role of functional testing, such as blood tests and other assessments, in understanding individual nutritional requirements and addressing deficiencies.

Implementing Personalized Nutrition Strategies

- **Dietary Modifications:**
Providing insights into modifying dietary choices based on individual needs, preferences, and health goals, tailoring macronutrient ratios, and food selection.

- **Meal Planning and Tracking:**
Discussing the use of meal planning apps, tracking tools, and professional guidance to support personalized nutrition goals.

Embracing Personalized Nutrition for Longevity

Understanding the importance of personalized nutrition empowers individuals to make informed dietary choices that cater to their unique needs and goals. By adopting personalized approaches to nutrition, individuals can optimize their diets, support overall health, and potentially extend their health span by embracing dietary strategies that align with their individual profiles.

In the subsequent chapters, we'll continue our exploration, discussing additional lifestyle strategies and practical implementations for fostering a longer, healthier life through personalized nutrition and wellness practices.

CHAPTER 12

LONGEVITY MINDSET AND LIFESTYLE INTEGRATION

Cultivating Habits for a Healthier, More Fulfilling Life

Beyond nutrition and specific practices, cultivating a longevity mindset and integrating holistic lifestyle habits stand as integral components in the pursuit of a longer, healthier life. In this chapter, we'll explore the importance of mindset, habits, and holistic lifestyle integration in promoting overall well-being and longevity.

The Power of Mindset in Longevity

- **Positive Psychology:**

Exploring the impact of positive thinking, resilience, and optimism on health outcomes and their potential contribution to longevity.

- **Mindfulness Practices:**

Discuss mindfulness techniques, gratitude exercises, and their role in reducing stress, enhancing well-being, and supporting overall health.

Holistic Lifestyle Integration

- **Social Connections:**

Investigating the significance of social interactions, community engagement, and strong social connections in fostering emotional well-being and longevity.

- **Purpose and Fulfillment:**

Understanding the importance of having a sense of purpose, engaging in meaningful activities, and their potential impact on health and longevity.

Implementing Lifestyle Habits for Longevity

- Physical Activity Beyond Exercise:
Emphasizing the importance of daily movement, non-exercise activities, and staying active throughout the day for overall health.

- Nature and Outdoor Engagement:
Discussing the benefits of spending time in nature, connecting with the outdoors, and its potential impact on mental and physical well-being.

Embracing a Longevity-Focused Lifestyle

Recognizing the impact of mindset and holistic lifestyle integration on health and longevity empowers individuals to adopt habits that contribute to a healthier and more fulfilling life. By fostering positive attitudes, nurturing social connections, and embracing holistic lifestyle practices, individuals can optimize their well-being and potentially extend their health span.

In the subsequent chapters, we'll summarize and provide actionable insights from various aspects discussed, offering a comprehensive approach to nutrition, wellness, and lifestyle for longevity.

CHAPTER 13:
SUSTAINABLE PRACTICES FOR LONG-TERM HEALTH

Nurturing Consistency for Lasting Well-being

As we've explored various aspects of nutrition, metabolism, lifestyle integration, and mindset in the pursuit of longevity, this chapter aims to underscore the importance of sustainability in maintaining long-term health practices. It delves into fostering consistency, overcoming challenges, and sustaining healthy habits for enduring well-being.

Consistency in Healthy Habits

- Routine Formation:

Exploring the significance of creating consistent routines to solidify healthy habits, emphasizing regularity in meal patterns, exercise schedules, and self-care practices.

- **Mindful Persistence:**

Discussing the role of mindfulness in sustaining healthy behaviors, including staying present, setting realistic goals, and adapting to changes while maintaining focus on long-term health objectives.

Overcoming Roadblocks to Sustainability

- **Addressing Setbacks:**

Understanding that setbacks are part of the journey and providing strategies to overcome obstacles, bounce back from setbacks, and stay committed to health goals.

- **Maintaining Motivation:**

Discussing methods to stay motivated and inspired, including finding intrinsic motivators, seeking support networks, and celebrating small victories along the way.

Longevity in Lifestyle Integration

- Creating a Lifelong Approach:
Emphasizing the shift towards viewing health practices as a lifelong commitment rather than short-term endeavors fosters a sustainable and adaptive mindset.

- Flexibility and Adaptability:
Highlighting the importance of flexibility and adaptability in health habits, encouraging adjustments based on changing circumstances without compromising long-term goals.

Nurturing Lasting Well-being
Sustainability is the linchpin in the pursuit of lasting well-being. By nurturing consistency, resilience, and adaptability, individuals can transform intermittent efforts into lifelong practices, fostering enduring health, vitality, and a sustainable path toward a longer, healthier life.

In this final chapter, let us reaffirm our commitment to sustained health practices and embrace the journey towards lasting well-being—a journey marked not by temporary changes but by sustainable habits that promote vitality and a fulfilled life.

CONCLUSION

As we conclude this journey through the realms of nutrition, metabolism, lifestyle, and well-being, it becomes evident that the pursuit of longevity encompasses a multifaceted approach. The intricate interplay between nutrition, metabolic health, lifestyle habits, and mindset collectively shapes our potential for a longer, healthier life.

Throughout this book, we've explored the fundamental principles of nutrition, elucidated the complexities of metabolism and fat burning, and delved into the significance of micronutrients, superfoods, and personalized dietary approaches. We've discussed the roles of exercise, stress management, sleep quality, and the importance of mindset in fostering resilience and vitality.

Synergy of Lifestyle Factors: The synergy between these various lifestyle factors—nutrition, exercise, stress management, sleep, mindset, and holistic living—presents a comprehensive blueprint for longevity. It's not a singular element but the harmonious integration of these aspects that paves the way toward a longer, healthier life.

Empowerment Through Knowledge: Armed with knowledge, we've equipped ourselves to make informed choices, embracing a balanced diet rich in nutrients, incorporating regular physical activity, managing stress, prioritizing quality sleep, fostering a positive mindset, and integrating holistic lifestyle practices. These choices are the building blocks upon which a foundation for extended health span is constructed.

Individual Paths to Longevity: Recognizing that each individual's journey toward longevity is unique, we've explored varied approaches and strategies, emphasizing the importance of personalization and tailored choices that suit individual needs, genetic predispositions, and preferences.

Continuing the Journey: The pursuit of longevity is an ongoing journey—one that evolves with each decision, habit, and conscious effort toward health and wellness. It's about embracing a lifestyle that supports not only a longer lifespan but also a fuller, more vibrant life.

As we conclude this chapter, let this book serve as a guide—a roadmap that empowers you to navigate the intricacies of nutrition, metabolism, and lifestyle, steering you towards a path of enhanced health, vitality, and the potential for an extended health span.

Here's to your journey towards longevity, well-being, and thriving in the fullest sense of the word.